Low Carb

Step By Step Low Carb Diet For Beginners And Gluten Free Recipes On Low Carb Diet For Loss Weight

(Simple And Effective Low Carb Recipes For Weight Loss)

Louis Ross

Table Of Contents

Bacon Cheeseburger Waffles 1

Keto Breakfast Cheesecake 4

Fresh Egg   -Crust Pizza 7

Breakfast Roll-Ups 10

Basic Opie Rolls 12

Almond Coconut Fresh Egg   Wraps .. 14

Bacon & Avocado Omelet 15

Bacon & Cheese Frittata 17

Bacon & Fresh Egg   Breakfast Muffins
.... 18

Bacon Hash 20

Bagels With Cheese 22

Baked Apples 24

Baked Fresh Fresh Egg In The Avocado 25

Banana Pancakes 27

Breakfast Skillet 28

Simple Kimchi 29

Oven-Fried Green Beans 31

Cauliflower Mash 32

Portobello Mushrooms 33

Broiled Brussels Sprouts............................. 34

Pesto... 36

Brussels Sprouts And Bacon 37

Creamy Spinach 39

Avocado Fries 40

Roasted Cauliflower 42

Mushrooms And Spinach 43

Okra And Fresh Tomato   Es 45

Snap Peas And Mint..................................... 47

Collard Greens With Turkey 48

Fresh Egg   Plant And Fresh Tomatoes
.... 50

Taco Stuffed Avocados 52

- Buffalo Shrimp Lettuce Wraps 54
- Keto Bacon Sushi 56
- Keto Burger Fat Bombs 58
- Keto Taco Cups 60
- Caprese Zoodles 63
- Zucchini Sushi 65
- Asian Chicken Lettuce Wraps 67
- Prosciutto And Mozzarella Bomb 70
- Ketofied Chick-Fil-A-Style Chicken 72
- Cheeseburger Fresh Tomato   Es 74
- Korma Curry 76
- Zucchini Bars 78
- Mushroom Soup 80
- Stuffed Portobello Mushrooms 82
- Lettuce Salad 84
- Fresh Onion   Soup 86
- Asparagus Salad 88
- Beef With Cabbage Noodles 90

Roast Beef And Mozzarella Plate 92

Beef And Broccoli 94

Garlic Herb Beef Roast 96

Sprouts Stir-Fry With Kale, Broccoli, And Beef... 98

Beef And Vegetable Skillet 100

Beef, Pepper And Green Beans Stir-Fry .. 102

Keto Cheesecakes 104

Keto Brownies 106

Raspberry And Coconut 108

Chocolate Pudding Delight...................... 110

Peanut Butter Fudge 111

Cinnamon Streusel Fresh Egg   Loaf 113

Snickerdoodle Muffins 115

Yogurt And Strawberry Bowl 117

Sweet Cinnamon Muffin........................... 118

Nutty Muffins 119

Pumpkin And Cream Cheese Cup 120

Berries In Yogurt Cream 123

Pumpkin Pie Mug Cake 124

Chocolate And Strawberry Crepe 126

Blackberry And Coconut Flour Cupcake . 128

Coconut Soup 130

Broccoli Soup 132

Simple Fresh Tomato   Soup 134

Green Soup 136

Sausage And Peppers Soup 138

Avocado Soup 140

Avocado And Bacon Soup 142

Roasted Bell Peppers Soup 144

Spicy Bacon Soup 146

Italian Sausage Soup 148

Cabbage Hash Browns 150

Cauliflower Hash Browns 152

Bacon Cheeseburger Waffles

Ingredients:

- 6 tablespoons of parmesan cheese, grated
- 6 tablespoons of almond flour
- 2 teaspoon of fresh onion powder
- 2 teaspoon of garlic powder
- 2 cup (4 00 g) of cauliflower crumbles
- 2 fresh fresh egg s
- 6 ounces of cheddar cheese
- 6 ounces of cheddar cheese
- 6 tablespoons of sugar-free barbecue sauce
- 6 slices of bacon
- 6 ounces of ground beef, 8 0% lean meat and 6 0% fat
- Waffle dough
- Pepper and salt to taste

Directions

1. Shred about 6 ounces of cheddar cheese, then add in cauliflower crumbles in a bowl and put in 2 of the cheddar cheese.
2. Put into the mixture spices, almond flour, fresh fresh fresh egg s and parmesan cheese, then mix and put aside for some time.
3. Thinly slice the bacon and cook in a skillet on medium to high heat.
4. After the bacon is cooked partially, put in the beef, cook until the mixture is well done.
5. Then put the excess grease from the bacon mixture into the waffle mixture. Set aside the bacon mix.
6. Use an immersion blender to blend the waffle mix until it becomes a paste, then add into the waffle iron 2 of the mix and cook until it becomes crispy.

7. Repeat for the remaining waffle mixture.
8. As the waffles cook, add sugar-free barbecue sauce to the ground beef and bacon mixture in the skillet.
9. Then proceed to assemble waffles by topping them with 2 of the left cheddar cheese and 2 the beef mixture. Repeat this for the remaining waffles, broil for around 2 0-2 6 minutes until the cheese has melted then serve right away.

Keto Breakfast Cheesecake

Ingredients

Toppings

- 4   cup of sweetener
- 6 fresh fresh egg   s
- 8 ounces of cream cheese
- 2 ounces of cottage cheese
- Crust ingredients
- 6   tablespoons of salted butter
- 2 tablespoons of sweetener
- 2 cups of almonds, whole
- cup of mixed berries for each cheesecake, frozen and thawed
- Filling ingredients
- 2 teaspoon of vanilla extract
- 2 teaspoon of almond extract

Directions

1. Preheat oven to around 680 degrees F.
2. Pulse almonds in a food processor then add in butter and sweetener.
3. Pulse until all the ingredients mix well and coarse dough forms.
4. Coat twelve silicone muffin pans using foil or paper liners.
5. Divide the batter evenly between the muffin pans then press into the bottom part until it forms a crust and bakes for about 8 minutes.
6. In the meantime, mix in a food processor the cream cheese and cottage cheese then pulse until the mixture is smooth.
7. Put in the extracts and sweetener then combine until well mixed.
8. Add in fresh fresh eggs and pulse again until it becomes smooth; you might need to scrape down the mixture from the sides of the processor. Share equally the batter between the muffin

pans, then bake for around 60-66 minutes until the middle is not wobbly when you shake the muffin pan lightly.
9. Put aside until cooled completely, then put in the refrigerator for about 2-2 ½ hours and then top with frozen and thawed berries.

Fresh Egg -Crust Pizza

Ingredients

- 2 fresh fresh fresh egg   s beaten well
- 6 teaspoons of olive oil
- 2 teaspoon of dried oregano to taste
- 2 teaspoon of spike seasoning to taste
- 2   ounce of mozzarella, chopped into small cubes
- 2   sliced thinly black olives
- 6 slices of turkey pepperoni, sliced into 2

- 6 thinly sliced small grape fresh tomato es

Directions

1 Preheat the broiler in an oven than in a small bowl, beat well the fresh fresh egg

s. Cut the pepperoni and fresh tomatoes in slices then cut the mozzarella cheese into cubes.

2. Put some olive oil in a skillet over medium heat, then heat the pan for around one minute until it begins to get hot. Add in fresh fresh eggs and season with oregano and spike seasoning, then cook for around 10 minutes until the fresh fresh eggs begin to set at the bottom.

3. Drizzle 2 of the mozzarella, olives, pepperoni, and fresh tomatoes on the fresh fresh eggs followed by another layer of the remaining 2 of the above ingredients. Ensure that there is a lot of cheese on the topmost layers. Cover the skillet using a lid and cook until the cheese begins to melt and the fresh fresh eggs are set, for around 20-26 minutes.

4. Place the pan under the preheated broiler and cook until the top has

browned and the cheese has melted nicely for around 20-25 minutes. Serve immediately.

Breakfast Roll-Ups

Ingredients

- 6 slices of cooked bacon
- 6 cups of cheddar cheese, shredded
- Pepper and salt
- 2   fresh   fresh fresh egg   s
- Non-stick cooking spray
- 6 patties of cooked breakfast sausage

Directions

1. Preheat a skillet on medium to high heat, then using a whisk, combine two of the fresh fresh egg   s in a mixing bowl.
2. After the pan has become hot, lower the heat to medium-low heat then put in the fresh fresh egg   s . If you want to, you can utilize some cooking spray.
3. Season fresh fresh egg   s with some pepper and salt.

4. Cover the fresh fresh eggs and leave them to cook for a couple of minutes or until the fresh fresh eggs are almost cooked.
5. Drizzle around 2 cup of cheese on top of the fresh fresh fresh eggs then place a strip of bacon and divide the sausage into two and place on top.
6. Roll the fresh egg carefully on top of the fillings. The roll-up will almost look like a taquito. If you have a hard time folding over the fresh egg, use a spatula to keep the fresh egg intact until the fresh egg has molded into a roll-up.
7. Put aside the roll-up then repeat the above steps until you have four more roll-ups; you should have 6 roll-ups in total.

Basic Opie Rolls

Ingredients

- 6 ounces of cream cheese
- 6 fresh fresh egg
- 2 teaspoon of salt
- 2 teaspoon of cream of tartar

Directions

1. Preheat the oven to about 625 degrees F, then separate the fresh egg whites from fresh egg yolks and place both fresh fresh egg s in different bowls. Using an electric mixer, beat well the fresh egg whites until the mixture is very bubbly, then add in the cream of tartar and mix again until it forms a stiff peak.

2. In the bowl with the fresh egg yolks, put in 6 ounces of cubed cheese and salt. Mix well until the mixture has doubled in size and is pale yellow. Put in the fresh egg white mixture into the fresh egg yolk mixture then fold the mixture gently together.
3. Spray some oil on the cookie sheet coated with some parchment paper, then add dollops of the batter and bake for around 8 0 minutes.
4. You will know they are ready when the upper part of the rolls is firm and golden. Leave them to cool for a few minutes on a wire rack. Enjoy with some coffee.

Almond Coconut Fresh Egg Wraps

Ingredients:

- 4 6 tsp Sea salt
- 2 tbsp almond meal
- 6 Organic fresh fresh eggs
- 2 tbsp Coconut flour

Directions:

1. Combine the fixings in a blender and work them until creamy. Heat a skillet using the med-high temperature setting.
2. Pour two tablespoons of batter into the skillet and cook - covered about three minutes. Turn it over to cook for another 2 0 minutes.
3. Serve the wraps piping hot.

Bacon & Avocado Omelet

Ingredients:

- 6 cup freshly grated parmesan cheese
- 2 tbsp Ghee or coconut oil or butter
- 2 of 2 small Avocado
- 2 slice Crispy bacon
- 2 Fresh   organic fresh fresh egg   s

Directions:

1. Prepare the bacon to your liking and set aside. Combine the fresh fresh fresh egg s parmesan cheese, and your choice of finely chopped herbs. Warm a skillet and add the butter/ghee to melt using the medium-high heat setting. When the pan is hot, whisk and add the fresh fresh egg s .

2. Prepare the omelet working it towards the middle of the pan for about 8 6 seconds. When firm, flip, and cook it for another 8 6 seconds.
3. Arrange the omelet on a plate and garnish with the crunched bacon bits.
4. Serve with sliced avocado.

Bacon & Cheese Frittata

Ingredients:

- 2 cup Heavy cream
- 6 Fresh fresh egg   s
- 6 Crispy slices of bacon
- 2 Chopped green onions
- 2 oz Cheddar cheese
- Also Needed: 2 pie plate

Directions:

1. Warm the oven temperature to reach 610 0 º Fahrenheit.
2. Whisk the fresh fresh egg   s and seasonings. Empty into the pie pan and top off with the remainder of the fixings. Bake 60-8 0 minutes. Wait for a few minutes before serving for best results.

Bacon & Fresh Egg Breakfast Muffins

Ingredients:

- 8 slices Bacon
- 2 cup Green fresh onion
- 8 fresh fresh egg   s

Directions:

1. Warm the oven at 680 ° Fahrenheit. Spritz the muffin tin wells using a cooking oil spray. Chop the onions and set aside.
2. Prepare a fresh skillet using the medium temperature setting. Fry the bacon until it's crispy and place on a layer of paper towels to drain the grease.

3. Chop it into small pieces after it has cooled.
4. Whisk the fresh fresh fresh egg s bacon, and green fresh onions, mixing well until all of the fixings are incorporated. Dump the fresh egg mixture into the muffin tin (2 way full). Bake it for about 26 to 4 0 minutes. Cool slightly and serve.

Bacon Hash

Ingredients:

6   Fresh fresh egg   s

6 Bacon slices

2 Small green pepper

2 Jalapenos

2 Small onion

Directions:

1. Chop the bacon into chunks using a food processor. Set aside for now. Slice the onions and peppers into thin strips. Dice the jalapenos as small as possible.
2. Heat a skillet and fry the vfresh egg ies. Once browned, combine the fixings and cook until crispy. Place on a serving dish with the fresh fresh egg   s .

Bagels With Cheese

Ingredients:

- 2 Fresh fresh egg   s
- 6 cups Mozzarella cheese
- 2 tsp. Baking powder
- 6 oz Cream cheese
- 6 cups Almond flour

Directions:

1. Shred the mozzarella and combine with the flour, baking powder, and cream cheese in a mixing container.
2. Pop into the microwave for about one minute.
3. Mix well.
4. Let the mixture cool and add the fresh fresh egg   s . Break apart into8 sections and shape into round bagels.

Note: You can also sprinkle with a seasoning of your choice or pinch of salt if desired.
5. Bake them for approximately 4 0 to 4 6 minutes.
6. Serve or cool and store.

Baked Apples

Ingredients:

- 2 .6 cup chopped pecans
- 6 fresh Granny Smith apples
- 6 tsp Keto-friendly sweetener.
- 2 tsp Cinnamon

Directions:

1. Set the oven temperature at 8 00 ° Fahrenheit. Mix the sweetener with the cinnamon and pecans.
2. Core the apple and add the prepared stuffing.
3. Add enough water into the baking dish to cover the bottom of the apple. Bake them for about 2 10 minutes to 2-2 ½ hour.

Baked Fresh Fresh Egg In The Avocado

Ingredients:

- 2 of 2 Avocado
- 2 Fresh egg
- 2 tbsp Olive oil
- 2 cup shredded cheddar cheese

Directions:

1 Heat the oven to reach 640 ° Fahrenheit.
2 Discard the avocado pit and remove just enough of the 'insides' to add the fresh egg . Drizzle with oil and break the fresh egg into the shell.
3 Sprinkle with cheese and bake them for 4 0 to 40 minutes until the fresh egg is the way you prefer. Serve.

Banana Pancakes

Ingredients:

- 6 Fresh fresh egg   s
- 2 tsp Cinnamon
- 2 tsp Baking powder (Optional)
- Butter
- 2 Bananas

Directions:

1. Combine each of the fixings. Melt a portion of butter in a skillet using the medium temperature setting.
2. Prepare the pancakes 2 0-2 6   minutes per side. Cook them with the lid on for the first part of the cooking cycle for a fluffier pancake.

3. Serve plain or with your favorite garnishes such as a dollop of coconut cream or fresh berries.

Breakfast Skillet

Ingredients:

- 6 Organic fresh fresh eggs
- 2 cup Keto-friendly salsa of choice
- 2 lb. Organic ground turkey/grass-fed beef

Directions:

1. Warm the skillet using oil (medium heat). Add the turkey and simmer until the pink is gone. Fold in the salsa and simmer for two to three minutes.
2. Crack the fresh fresh eggs and add to the top of the turkey base. Place a lid on the pot and cook for seven minutes

until the whites of the fresh fresh eggs are opaque.

Simple Kimchi

Ingredients:

- tablespoons salt
- 2 pound napa cabbage, chopped
- 2 carrot, julienned
- 2 cup daikon radish
- green fresh onion   stalks, chopped
- 2 tablespoon fish sauce
- tablespoons chili flakes
- garlic cloves, peeled and minced
- 2 tablespoon sesame oil
- inch fresh ginger, peeled and grated

Directions:

1. In a bowl, mix the cabbage with the salt, massage well for 35minutes, cover, and set aside for 2-2 ½ hour.
2. In a bowl, mix the chili flakes with fish sauce, garlic, sesame oil, and ginger, and stir well.
3. Drain the cabbage well, rinse under cold water, and transfer to a bowl.
4. Add the carrots, green fresh onions, radish, and chili paste and stir.
5. Leave in a dark and cold place for at least 2 days before serving.

Oven-Fried Green Beans

Ingredients:

- 2 teaspoon paprika
- ⅔ Cup Parmesan cheese, grated
- 2 fresh fresh egg
- 35ounces green beans
- Salt and ground black pepper, to taste
- 2 teaspoon garlic powder

Directions:

1. In a bowl, mix the Parmesan cheese with salt, pepper, garlic powder, and paprika.
2. In another bowl, whisk the fresh egg with salt and pepper.
3. Dredge the green beans in fresh egg , and then in the Parmesan mixture. Place the green beans on a lined baking

sheet, place in an oven at 650ºF for 35 minutes.

Cauliflower Mash

Ingredients:

2 cup sour cream

2 small cauliflower head, separated into florets

Salt and ground black pepper, to taste

2 tablespoons feta cheese, crumbled

2 tablespoons black olives, pitted and sliced

Directions:

Put water in a pot, add some salt, bring to a boil over medium heat, add the florets, cook for 35minutes, take off the heat, and drain.

Return the cauliflower to the pot, add salt, black pepper, and sour cream, and blend using an immersion blender.

Add the black olives and feta cheese, stir and serve.

Portobello Mushrooms

Ingredients:

- 2 tablespoons balsamic vinegar
- 35ounces Portobello mushrooms, sliced
- Salt and ground black pepper, to taste
- 2 teaspoon dried basil
- 2 tablespoons olive oil
- 2 teaspoon tarragon, dried
- 2 teaspoon dried rosemary
- 2 teaspoon dried thyme

Directions:

1. In a bowl, mix the oil with vinegar, salt, pepper, rosemary, tarragon, basil, and thyme, and whisk.
2. Add the mushroom slices, toss to coat well, place them on a preheated grill over medium-high heat, cook for 10 minutes on both sides, and serve.

Broiled Brussels Sprouts

Ingredients:

- 2 pound Brussels sprouts, trimmed and halved
- Salt and ground black pepper, to taste
- 2 teaspoon sesame seeds
- 2 tablespoon green fresh onions, chopped
- 35 tablespoons sukrin gold syrup

- 2 tablespoon coconut aminos
- 2 tablespoons sesame oil
- 2 tablespoon sriracha

Directions:

1. In a bowl, mix the sesame oil with coconut aminos, sriracha, syrup, salt, and black pepper, and whisk.
2. Heat a pan over medium-high heat, add the Brussels sprouts, and cook them for 10 minutes on each side.
3. Add the sesame oil mixture, toss to coat, sprinkle sesame seeds, and green fresh onions, stir again, and serve.

Pesto

Ingredients:

- 2 cup Parmesan cheese, grated
- 2 garlic cloves, peeled and chopped
- Salt and ground black pepper, to taste
- cup olive oil
- 2 cups basil
- 2 cup pine nuts

Directions:

1. Put the basil in a food processor, add the pine nuts, and garlic, and blend well.
2. Add the Parmesan cheese, salt, pepper, and the oil gradually and blend again until you obtain a paste.
3. Serve with chicken or vegetables.

Brussels Sprouts And Bacon

Ingredients:

- Salt and ground black pepper, to taste
- A pinch of cumin
- A pinch of red pepper, crushed
- 2 tablespoons extra virgin olive oil
- 8 bacon strips, chopped
- pound Brussels sprouts, trimmed and halved

Directions:

1 In a bowl, mix the Brussels sprouts with salt, pepper, cumin, red pepper, and oil, and toss to coat.
2 Spread the Brussels sprouts on a lined baking sheet, place in an oven at 700 ºF, and bake for 85   minutes.

3 Heat a pan over medium heat, add the bacon pieces, and cook them until they become crispy.
4 Divide the baked Brussels sprouts on plates, top with bacon, and serve.

Creamy Spinach

Ingredients:

- Salt and ground black pepper, to taste
- tablespoons sour cream
- 2 tablespoon butter
- 2 tablespoons Parmesan cheese, grated
- 2 garlic cloves, peeled and minced
- 8 ounces of spinach leaves
- A drizzle of olive oil

Directions:

1. Heat a pan with the oil over medium heat, add the spinach, stir and cook until it softens.
2. Add the salt, pepper, butter, Parmesan cheese, and butter, stir, and cook for 8 minutes.

3. Add the sour cream, stir, and cook for 20 minutes.
4. Divide between plates and serve.

Avocado Fries

Ingredients:

- 35 cups almond meal
- A pinch of cayenne pepper
- Salt and ground black pepper, to taste
- 6 avocados, pitted, peeled, halved, and sliced
- 35 cups sunflower oil

Directions:

1 In a bowl, mix the almond meal with salt, pepper, and cayenne, and stir. In a second bowl, whisk fresh fresh eggs with a pinch of salt and pepper.

2. Dredge the avocado pieces in fresh egg and then in almond meal mixture. Heat a pan with the oil over medium-high heat, add the avocado fries, and cook them until they are golden.
3. Transfer to paper towels, drain grease, and divide between plates and serve.

Roasted Cauliflower

Ingredients:

- 2 tablespoons extra virgin olive oil
- 2 cauliflower head, separated into florets
- Salt and ground black pepper, to taste
- 2 cup Parmesan cheese, grated
- 2 tablespoon fresh parsley, chopped
- 6 tablespoons olive oil

Directions:

1. In a bowl, mix the oil with garlic, salt, pepper, and cauliflower florets.
2. Toss to coat well, spread this on a lined baking sheet, place in an oven at 850 ºF, and bake for 4 0 minutes, stirring 2 way. Add the Parmesan cheese, and parsley, stir and cook for 2 0 minutes.

3 Divide between plates and serve.

Mushrooms And Spinach

Ingredients:

- 2 cup fresh parsley, chopped
- 2 onion, peeled and chopped
- 6 tablespoons olive oil
- 2 tablespoons balsamic vinegar
- 2 ounces spinach leaves, chopped
- Salt and ground black pepper, to taste
- 3 ounces mushrooms, chopped
- 2 garlic cloves, peeled and minced

Directions:

1 Heat a pan with the oil over medium-high heat, add the garlic and onion, stir, and cook for 8 minutes.

2. Add the mushrooms, stir, and cook for 6 minutes.
3. Add the spinach, stir, and cook for 6 minutes.
4. Add the vinegar, salt, and pepper, stir, and cook for 2 minute.
5. Add the parsley, stir, divide between plates, and serve.

Okra And Fresh Tomato Es

Ingredients:

- 2 onion, peeled and chopped
- 2 pound okra, trimmed and sliced
- 2 bacon slices, chopped
- 2 small green bell peppers, seeded and chopped
- 4ounces canned stewed fresh tomato es, cored and chopped
- 2 Salt and ground black pepper, to taste
- 2 celery stalks, chopped

Directions:

1 Heat a pan over medium-high heat, add the bacon, stir, brown for a few minutes, transfer to paper towels, and set aside. Heat the pan again over medium heat,

add the okra, bell pepper, onion, and celery, stir, and cook for 6 minutes.
2. Add the fresh tomatoes, salt, and pepper, stir, and cook for 6 minutes.
3. Divide between plates, garnish with crispy bacon, and serve.

Snap Peas And Mint

Ingredients:

- 2 tablespoon mint leaves, chopped
- 2 teaspoons olive oil
- 6 green fresh onions, chopped
- 2 garlic clove, peeled and minced
- 1/2 pound sugar snap peas, trimmed
- Salt and ground black pepper, to taste

Directions:

1. Heat a pan with the oil over medium-high heat.
2. Add the snap peas, salt, pepper, green fresh onions, garlic, and mint.
3. Stir everything, cook for 6 minutes, divide between plates, and serve.

Collard Greens With Turkey

Ingredients:

- 6 cups chicken stock
- 2 turkey leg
- 2 tablespoons garlic, minced
- 2 cup olive oil
- 6 bunches collard greens, chopped
- Salt and ground black pepper, to taste
- 2 tablespoon red pepper flakes

Directions:

1. Heat a pot with the oil over medium heat, add the garlic, stir, and cook for 2 minute.
2. Add the stock, salt, pepper, and turkey leg stir, cover, and simmer for 8 0 minutes.

3   Add the collard greens, cover pot again, and cook for 6 20 minutes.
4   Reduce heat to medium, add more salt and pepper, stir, and cook for 2 hour.
5   Drain the greens, chop up the turkey, mix everything with the red pepper flakes, stir, divide between plates, and serve.

Fresh Egg Plant And Fresh Tomatoes

Ingredients:

- Salt and ground black pepper, to taste
- 2 cup Parmesan cheese, grated
- A drizzle of olive oil
- 2 fresh tomato, sliced
- 2 fresh egg plant, sliced into thin rounds

Directions:

1. Place fresh egg plant slices on a lined baking dish, drizzle some oil and sprinkle 2 of the Parmesan.
2. Top fresh egg plant slices with fresh tomato ones, season with some salt and pepper, and sprinkle the rest of the cheese over them.

3. Place in an oven at 6 00ºF, and bake for 2 2 0 minutes.
4. Divide between plates and serve hot as a side dish.

Taco Stuffed Avocados

Ingredients:

- 2 Packet Taco Seasoning
- Kosher Salt
- Freshly Ground Black Pepper
- 2 Cup Shredded Mexican Cheese
- 2 Cup Shredded Lettuce
- 2 Cup Quartered Grape Fresh tomatoes
- Sour cream, for topping
- 6 Ripe Avocados
- 2 Juice of 2 Lime
- 2 Tbsp. Extra-Virgin Olive Oil
- 2 Medium Onion, Chopped
- 2 Lb. Ground Beef

Directions:

1. Pit and halve the avocados.
2. With a scoop, scoop out a bit of avocado flesh to create a hole.
3. Dice the removed avocado fresh and set aside for later.
4. Pour lime juice over the avocados to prevent browning.
5. Heat oil in a preheated skillet over medium heat and add chopped onion.
6. Cook the fresh onion until translucent for 6 -6 minutes.
7. Stir in ground beef and taco seasoning, breaking up the meat with a wooden spoon.
8. Season the beef with salt and pepper, cook until the meat is browned and no longer pink, about 6 minutes.
9. Turn off the heat and drain the fat, top each avocado 2 with the cooked beef mixture.

Buffalo Shrimp Lettuce Wraps

Ingredients:

- Freshly Ground Black Pepper
- 2 Head Romaine lettuce, Leaves Separated, For Serving
- 2 Red Onion, Finely Chopped
- 2 Rib Celery, Sliced Thin
- 2 C. Blue Cheese, Crumbled
- 2 Tbsp. Butter
- 2 Garlic Cloves, Minced
- 1 Hot Sauce, Such as Frank's
- 2 Tbsp. Extra-Virgin Olive Oil
- Lb. Shrimp, Peeled and Deveined, Tails Removed
- Kosher Salt

Directions:

1. Make buffalo sauce: In a saucepan over medium heat, melt butter. When melted completely, put garlic and cook until fragrant, about 2 minute. Put hot sauce and stir to combine—reduce to low when you cook the shrimp.
2. Make shrimp: In a big skillet over medium heat, heat oil. Put shrimp and season with salt and pepper. Cook, flipping 2 way through, until opaque, about two minutes per side. Turn off heat and put the buffalo sauce, tossing to coat.
3. Assemble wraps: Put a tiny of shrimp mixture to the center of a romaine leaf. Then top with red onion, celery, and blue cheese.

Keto Bacon Sushi

Ingredients:

- 2 medium carrots, thinly sliced
- 2 avocado, sliced
- 6 oz. cream cheese softened
- Sesame seeds, for garnish
- 6 slices bacon, halved
- 2 Persian cucumbers, thinly sliced

Directions:

1. Heat oven to 850 °F (206 °C), line a baking tray with aluminum foil and fit it with a cooling rack.
2. Lay bacon halves in an even layer on the lined baking sheet and place in the oven.
3. Bake until lightly crunchy but still pliable, about 35 to 40 minutes.

4. In the meantime, cut cucumbers, carrots, and avocado into pieces roughly the width of the bacon.
5. Once the bacon is cool enough to touch, spread an even layer of cream cheese on each slice.
6. Divide vegetables evenly between the bacon and place on one end.
7. Roll up vegetables tightly.
8. Garnish with sesame seeds and serve.
9. Enjoy!

Keto Burger Fat Bombs

Ingredients:

- 2 tbsp. cold butter, cut into 25 pieces
- 2 oz. cheddar, cut into 25 pieces
- Lettuce leaves, for serving
- Thinly sliced fresh tomatoes, for serving
- Mustard, for serving
- 2 lb. ground beef
- 2 tsp. garlic powder
- Kosher salt
- Freshly ground black pepper

Directions:

1 Heat oven to 600 °F (2 2 0 0 °C), grease a mini muffin tin with cooking spray.

2. In a medium bowl, season beef with garlic powder, salt, and pepper.
3. Press one teaspoon beef consistently into the bottom of each muffin tin cup, totally covering the bottom.
4. Place a slice of butter on top then press one teaspoon beef over butter to cover.
5. Place a slice of cheddar on top of meat in each cup then press remaining beef over cheese to cover.
6. Bake the fat bombs until meat is golden and cook through for about 2 6 minutes.
7. Let cool slightly.
8. Carefully, use a metal offset spatula to release each burger from the tin. Serve with lettuce leaves, fresh tomato es, and mustard.
9. Enjoy!

Keto Taco Cups

Ingredients:

- 2 Tbsp. Extra-Virgin Olive Oil
- 2 Small Onion, Chopped
- Kosher salt
- Freshly ground black pepper
- Sour cream, for serving
- Diced avocado, for serving
- Freshly chopped cilantro, for serving
- Chopped fresh tomato   es, for serving
- 6 Cloves Garlic, Minced
- 2 Lb. Ground Beef
- 2 Tsp. Chili Powder
- 2 Tsp. Ground Cumin
- 2 Tsp. Paprika
- Shredded Cheddar

Directions:

1. Preheat oven to 650°F (2 2 0 0 °C).
2. Line a fresh baking tray with parchment paper or a baking mat.
3. Put about 2 tablespoons cheddar with a space of 2-inches.
4. Bake the cheese until bubbly and edges turn to golden, about 6 -8 minutes.
5. Let the crisps cool on the baking sheet for a minute.
6. Grease bottom of a muffin tin with cooking spray set aside.
7. Put the backed melted cheese slices on the bottom of a muffin tin.
8. Top with another muffin tin and let it cool for 8-35minutes.
9. Heat oil in a skillet over medium heat, add chopped fresh onion and cook until soft.
10. Add garlic and cook until fragrant, add ground beef, breaking up meat with a spatula.

11 Cook until beef is browned and no longer pink, about 6 -6 minutes, then drain the fat.
12 Add meat again to the skillet and season with chili powder, cumin, paprika, salt, and pepper.
13 Place cheese cups on a serving platter.
14 Fill the cheese cups with cooked ground beef and top with sour cream, avocado, cilantro, and fresh tomatoes.
15 Enjoy!

Caprese Zoodles

Ingredients:

- 4 Cherry Fresh tomato   es Halved
- 2 C. Mozzarella Balls, Quartered If Fresh
- Fresh Basil Leaves
- 1 Tbsp. Balsamic Vinegar
- 6   Fresh   Zucchini
- 2 Tbsp. Extra-Virgin Olive Oil
- 1 Kosher Salt
- Freshly Ground Black Pepper

Directions:

1. Using a spiralizer, make zoodles out of zucchini.
2. Put zoodles to a big bowl, toss with olive oil and season with pepper and salt.
3. Let marinate 2 6 minutes.

4. Combine in fresh tomato es, mozzarella, and basil to zoodles in a bowl and toss until combined.
5. . Drizzle with balsamic and serve.
6. Enjoy!

Zucchini Sushi

Ingredients:

- 2 c. lump crab meat
- 2 carrot, cut into thin matchsticks
- 2 avocado, diced
- 2 cucumber, cut into thin matchsticks
- 2 tsp. toasted sesame seeds
- 2 medium zucchini
- 6 oz. cream cheese softened
- 2 tsp. Sriracha hot sauce
- 2 tsp. lime juice

Directions:

1 With a vegetable peeler, slice each zucchini into even thin strips.
2 Place zucchini on a lined plate to dry up the moisture.

3. In a bowl, whisk together cream cheese, Sriracha, and lime juice.
4. Place two zucchini slices down straight on a cutting board.
5. Top with cream cheese in a thin layer on the lift side top with crab, cucumber, and avocado.
6. Roll the zucchini tightly from the lift side.
7. Repeat the process with the remaining zucchini pieces.
8. Garnish with sesame seeds before serving.

Asian Chicken Lettuce Wraps

Ingredients:

- 2 cloves garlic, minced
- 2 tbsp. freshly grated ginger
- 2 lb. ground chicken
- 2 c. water chestnuts, drained and sliced
- 2 green fresh onions, thinly sliced
- Kosher salt
- Freshly ground black pepper
- Fresh leafy lettuce (leaves separated), for serving
- 6 tbsp. hoisin sauce
- 2 tbsp. low-sodium soy sauce
- 2 tbsp. rice wine vinegar
- 2 tbsp. Sriracha (optional)
- 2 tsp. sesame oil
- 2 tbsp. extra-virgin olive oil
- 2 medium onion, diced

Directions:

1. Make the sauce: In a thin bowl.
2. Whisk together hoisin sauce, rice wine vinegar, soy sauce, Sriracha, and sesame oil.
3. In a big skillet over medium-high heat, preheat olive oil.
4. Put onions and cook until soft, about 6 minutes.
5. Then stir in garlic and ginger and cook until fragrant, about 2 minute more.
6. Put ground chicken and cook until opaque and typically cooked through, breaking up meat with a wooden spoon.
7. Pour in the sauce and cook 5 to 10 minutes more, until sauce reduces slightly and chicken cooked through thoroughly.
8. Turn off heat and stir in chestnuts and green onions.
9. Season with pepper and salt.

10 Spoon rice, if using, and a fresh scoop (about 2 cup) of chicken mixture into the center of each lettuce leaf. Serve immediately.

Prosciutto And Mozzarella Bomb

Ingredients:

- 8 oz (250g) fresh mozzarella ball
- Olive oil, for frying
- 6 oz (300g) sliced prosciutto

Directions:

1. Coating 2 of the prosciutto slices vertically.
2. Lay the remaining slices horizontally across the first set of slices.
3. Place your mozzarella ball, upside down, onto the crisscrossed prosciutto slices.
4. Firmly, but very carefully, wrap the mozzarella ball with the prosciutto slices.
5. If making ahead, wrap the balls in cling film and refrigerate.

6 To serve, heat the olive oil in a skillet and crisp the prosciutto on all sides.
7 Enjoy!

Ketofied Chick-Fil-A-Style Chicken

Ingredients:

- 2 cup grated Parmesan
- Salt and pepper, to taste
- 2 tsp paprika
- 2 fresh fresh fresh eggs
- 2 tbsp avocado oil
- 5 oz (680g) pickle jar
- 8 medium uncooked chicken breast tenders
- 6 tbsp almond flour

Directions:

1. In a plastic resealable bag, add the chicken and the pickle juice, marinate in the fridge
2. For 30 to 50 minutes.

3. On a plate combine the almond flour, grated Parmesan, salt, pepper, and paprika.
4. Whip the fresh fresh eggs together in a separate bowl.
5. Preheat a skillet over medium-high heat and heat the avocado oil.
6. First, dip the chicken pieces in the beaten fresh egg then place it in the breading mixture to coat.
7. Place the chicken into the skillet and cook until golden browned.

Cheeseburger Fresh Tomato Es

Ingredients:

- 2 tbsp. extra-virgin olive oil
- 2 medium onion, chopped
- 2 cloves garlic, minced
- 2 lb. ground beef
- 2 tbsp. ketchup
- 2 tbsp. yellow mustard
- 6 slicing fresh tomato es
- Kosher salt
- Freshly ground black pepper
- 1 shredded cheddar
- 1 shredded iceberg lettuce
- pickle coins
- 6 Sesame seeds, for garnish

Directions:

1. In a skillet over medium heat, heat oil.
2. Put fresh onion and cook until tender, about 6 minutes, then stir in garlic.
3. Place ground beef, cook and break up the meat with a spatula, cook until the beef browned about 6 minutes, drain fat.
4. Season with salt and pepper, then add the ketchup and mustard.
5. Flip fresh tomatoes so they are stem-side down.
6. Cut the fresh tomatoes into 8 wedges, being careful not to cut entirely through the fresh tomatoes.
7. Carefully spread open the wedges.
8. Divide cooked ground beef evenly among the fresh tomatoes.
9. Then top each with cheese and lettuce.
10. Garnish with pickle coins and sesame seeds.
11. Serve it and enjoy it!

Korma Curry

Ingredients:

- 2 teaspoon ground coriander
- 1/2   teaspoon ground cardamom
- 2 teaspoon ginger powder
- 2 teaspoon cayenne pepper
- 1/2   teaspoon ground cinnamon
- 2 fresh tomato , diced
- 2 teaspoon avocado oil
- 2 cup of water
- 6 pound chicken breast, skinless, boneless
- 2 teaspoon garam masala
- 2 teaspoon curry powder
- 2 tablespoon apple cider vinegar
- 2 coconut cream
- 2 cup organic almond milk

Directions:

1. Chop the chicken breast and put it in the saucepan.
2. Add avocado oil and start to cook it over the medium heat.
3. Sprinkle the chicken with garam masala, curry powder, apple cider vinegar, ground coriander, cardamom, ginger powder, cayenne pepper, ground cinnamon, and diced fresh tomato . Mix up the ingredients carefully. Cook them for 35 minutes.
4. Add water, coconut cream, and almond milk. Saute the meat for 35minutes more.

Zucchini Bars

Ingredients:

- 6 zucchini, grated
- 2 white onion, diced
- 2 teaspoons butter
- 6 fresh fresh fresh egg   s whisked
- 2 tablespoons coconut flour
- 2 teaspoon salt
- 2 teaspoon ground black pepper
- 6 oz goat cheese, crumbled
- 6 oz Swiss cheese, shredded
- 2 cup spinach, chopped
- 2 teaspoon baking powder
- 2 teaspoon lemon juice

Directions:

1 In the mixing bowl, mix up together grated zucchini, diced onion, fresh fresh

fresh egg s coconut flour, salt, ground black pepper, crumbled cheese, chopped spinach, baking powder, and lemon juice.
2 Add butter and churn the mixture until homogenous.
3 Line the baking dish with baking paper.
4 Transfer the zucchini mixture into the baking dish and flatten it.
5 Preheat the oven to 700 F and put the dish inside.
6 Cook it for 2 6 minutes. Then chill the meal well.
7 Cut it into bars.

Mushroom Soup

Ingredients:

- 2 white onion, diced
- 2 tablespoon butter
- 2 oz turnip, chopped
- 2 teaspoon dried dill
- 2 teaspoon ground black pepper
- 1/2 teaspoon smoked paprika
- 2 oz celery stalk, chopped
- 2 cup of water
- 2 cup of coconut milk
- 2 cup white mushrooms, chopped
- 2 carrot, chopped

Directions:

1 Pour water and coconut milk in the saucepan. Bring the liquid to boil.

2. Add chopped mushrooms, carrot, and turnip. Close the lid and boil for 35 minutes.
3. Meanwhile, put butter in the skillet. Add diced onion. Sprinkle it with dill, ground black pepper, and smoked paprika. Roast the fresh onion for 6 minutes.
4. Add the roasted fresh onion in the soup mixture.
5. Then add chopped celery stalk. Close the lid.
6. Cook soup for 35 minutes.
7. Then ladle it into the serving bowls.

Stuffed Portobello Mushrooms

Ingredients:

- 2 tablespoon cream cheese
- 2 teaspoon minced garlic
- 2 tablespoon fresh cilantro, chopped
- 6 oz Cheddar cheese, grated
- 2 teaspoon ground black pepper
- 2 tablespoons olive oil
- 2 teaspoon salt
- 2 portobello mushrooms
- 2 cup spinach, chopped, steamed
- 2 oz artichoke hearts, drained, chopped
- 2 tablespoon coconut cream

Directions:

1 Sprinkle mushrooms with olive oil and place in the tray.

2. Transfer the tray in the preheated to 660F oven and broil them for 20 minutes.
3. Meanwhile, blend artichoke hearts, coconut cream, cream cheese, minced garlic, and chopped cilantro.
4. Add grated cheese in the mixture and sprinkle with ground black pepper and salt.
5. Fill the broiled mushrooms with the cheese mixture and cook them for 10 minutes more. Serve the mushrooms only hot.

Lettuce Salad

Ingredients:

- 2 teaspoon sunflower seeds
- 2 teaspoon lemon juice
- 2 fresh egg, boiled, peeled
- 2 oz Cheddar cheese, shredded
- 2 cup Romaine lettuce, roughly chopped
- 6 oz seitan, chopped
- 2 tablespoon avocado oil

Directions:

1. Place lettuce in the salad bowl. Add chopped seitan and shredded cheese.
2. Then chop the fresh egg roughly and add in the salad bowl too.
3. Mix up together lemon juice with the avocado oil.

4 Sprinkle the salad with the oil mixture and sunflower seeds. Don't stir the salad before serving.

Fresh Onion Soup

Ingredients:

- 6 cups of water
- 2 cup heavy cream
- 2 teaspoon salt
- 2 teaspoon chili flakes
- 2 teaspoon garlic powder
- 2 cups white onion, diced
- 6 tablespoon butter
- 2 cup white mushrooms, chopped

Directions:

1. Put butter in the saucepan and melt it.
2. Add diced white onion, chili flakes, and garlic powder. Mix it up and saute for 35minutes over the medium-low heat.
3. Then add water, heavy cream, and chopped mushrooms. Close the lid.

4　Cook the soup for 2 10 minutes more.
5　Then blend the soup until you get the creamy texture. Ladle it in the bowls.

Asparagus Salad

Ingredients:

- 6 oz Feta cheese, crumbled
- 2 cup lettuce, chopped
- 2 tablespoon canola oil
- 2 teaspoon apple cider vinegar
- 2 fresh tomato , diced
- 2 oz asparagus
- 2 tablespoon olive oil
- 2 teaspoon white pepper

Directions:

1. Preheat the oven to 700 F.
2. Place asparagus in the tray, sprinkle with olive oil and white pepper and transfer in the preheated oven. Cook it for 25 minutes.

3. Meanwhile, put crumbled Feta in the salad bowl.
4. Add chopped lettuce and diced fresh tomato .
5. Sprinkle the ingredients with apple cider vinegar.
6. Chill the cooked asparagus to the room temperature and add in the salad.
7. Shake the salad gently before serving.

Beef With Cabbage Noodles

Ingredients

- 6 oz fresh tomato sauce
- 2 tsp minced garlic
- 2 cup of water
- 6 oz ground beef
- 2 cup chopped cabbage

Seasoning:

- 2 tsp Italian seasoning
- 2 tsp dried basil
- 2 tbsp coconut oil
- 2 tsp salt

Directions:

1 Take a skillet pan, place it over medium heat, add oil and when hot, add beef and

cook for 10 minutes until nicely browned.
2. Meanwhile, prepare the cabbage and, for it, slice the cabbage into thin shred.
3. When the beef has cooked, add garlic, season with salt, basil, and Italian seasoning, stir well and continue cooking for 10 minutes until beef has thoroughly cooked.
4. Pour in fresh tomato sauce and water, stir well and bring the mixture to boil.
5. Then reduce heat to medium-low level, add cabbage, stir well until well mixed and simmer for 6 to 10 minutes until cabbage is softened, covering the pan.
6. Uncover the pan and continue simmering the beef until most of the cooking liquid has evaporated.
7. Serve.

Roast Beef And Mozzarella Plate

Ingredients

- 2 avocado, pitted
- 2 oz mozzarella cheese, cubed
- 2 cup mayonnaise
- 6 slices of roast beef
- 2 ounce chopped lettuce

Seasoning:

- 2 tsp ground black pepper
- 2 tbsp avocado oil
- 2 tsp salt

Directions:

1. Scoop out flesh from avocado and divide it evenly between two plates.

2. Add slices of roast beef, lettuce, and cheese and then sprinkle with salt and black pepper.
3. Serve with avocado oil and mayonnaise.

Beef And Broccoli

Ingredients:

- 6 oz broccoli florets, chopped
- 2 tbsp avocado oil
- 2 tbsp butter, unsalted
- 6 slices of beef roast, cut into strips
- 2 scallion, chopped

Seasoning:

- 2 tbsp soy sauce
- 2 tbsp chicken broth
- 2 tsp salt
- 2 tsp ground black pepper

Directions:

1. Take a medium skillet pan, place it over medium heat, add oil and when hot, add beef strips and cook for 2 minutes until hot.

2. Transfer beef to a plate, add scallion to the pan, then add butter and cook for 10 minutes until tender.
3. Add remaining ingredients, stir until mixed, switch heat to the low level, and simmer for 5 to 10 minutes until broccoli is tender.
4. Return beef to the pan, stir until well combined and cook for 2 minute.
5. Serve.

Garlic Herb Beef Roast

Ingredients:

- 2 tsp dried thyme
- 2 tsp dried rosemary
- 2 tbsp butter, unsalted
- 6 slices of beef roast
- 2 tsp garlic powder

Seasoning:

- 2 tsp ground black pepper
- 2 tsp salt

Direction:

1. Prepare the spice mix and for this, take a small bowl, place garlic powder, thyme, rosemary, salt, and black pepper and then stir until mixed.

2. Sprinkle spice mix on the beef roast.
3. Take a medium skillet pan, place it over medium heat, add butter and when it melts, add beef roast and then cook for 6 to 8 minutes until golden brown and cooked.
4. Serve.

Sprouts Stir-Fry With Kale, Broccoli, And Beef

Ingredients:

- 6 oz broccoli florets
- 6 oz kale
- 2 tbsp butter, unsalted
- 2 tsp red pepper flakes
- 6 slices of beef roast, chopped
- 2 oz Brussels sprouts, halved

Seasoning:

- 2 tsp garlic powder
- 2 tsp salt
- 2 tsp ground black pepper

Directions:

1. Take a medium skillet pan, place it over medium heat, add 1/2 tbsp butter and when it melts, add broccoli florets and sprouts, sprinkle with garlic powder, and cook for 6 minutes.
2. Season vegetables with salt and red pepper flakes, add chopped beef, stir until mixed and continue cooking for 10 minutes until browned on one side.
3. Then add kale along with remaining butter, flip the vegetables and cook for 2 minutes until kale leaves wilts.
4. Serve.

Beef And Vegetable Skillet

Ingredients:

- 2 pound ground beef
- 2 slices of bacon, diced
- 2 oz chopped asparagus
- 6 oz spinach, chopped

Seasoning:

- 2 tsp salt
- 2 tsp ground black pepper
- 6 tbsp coconut oil
- 2 tsp dried thyme

Directions:

1 Take a skillet pan, place it over medium heat, add oil and when hot, add beef and

bacon and cook for 6 to 8 minutes until slightly browned.
2. Then add asparagus and spinach, sprinkle with thyme, stir well and cook for 8 to 35minutes until thoroughly cooked.
3. Season skillet with salt and black pepper and serve.

Beef, Pepper And Green Beans Stir-Fry

Ingredients:

- 2 oz chopped green bell pepper
- 6 oz green beans
- 6 tbsp grated cheddar cheese
- 6 oz ground beef

Seasoning:

- 2 tsp salt
- 2 tsp ground black pepper
- 2 tsp paprika

Directions:

1. Take a skillet pan, place it over medium heat, add ground beef and cook for 10 minutes until slightly browned.

2. Then add bell pepper and green beans, season with salt, paprika, and black pepper, stir well and continue cooking for 8 to 35minutes until beef and vegetables have cooked through.
3. Sprinkle cheddar cheese on top, then transfer pan under the broiler and cook for 2 minutes until cheese has melted and the top is golden brown. And serve.

Keto Cheesecakes

Ingredients:

For the cheesecakes:

- 6 tablespoons coffee
- 8 ounces cream cheese
- 2   cup swerve sweetener
- 2 tablespoons butter
- 2 tablespoon caramel syrup; sugar-free
- fresh fresh egg   s

For the frosting:

- 8 ounces mascarpone cheese; soft
- 6 tablespoons caramel syrup; sugar-free
- 2 tablespoons swerve
- 6 tablespoons butter

Directions:

1. In your blender, mix cream cheese with fresh fresh fresh egg s 2 tablespoons butter, coffee, 2 tablespoon caramel syrup, and 2 cup swerve. Pulse very well.
2. Spoon this into a cupcakes pan, introduce in the oven at 680 degrees F and bake for 2 10 minutes
3. Leave aside to cool down and then keep in the freezer for 6 hours
4. Meanwhile, in a bowl, mix 6 tablespoons butter with 6 tablespoons caramel syrup, 2 tablespoons swerve, and mascarpone cheese and blend well.
5. Spoon this over cheesecakes and serve them.

Keto Brownies

Ingredients:

- 6 fresh fresh eggs
- 2 teaspoons vanilla
- 6 ounces of cocoa powder
- 2 teaspoon baking powder
- 6 ounces coconut oil; melted
- 6 ounces cream cheese
- 6 tablespoons swerve sweetener

Directions:

1. In a blender, mix fresh fresh eggs with coconut oil, cocoa powder, baking powder, vanilla, cream cheese, and swerve. Stir using a mixer.
2. Pour this into a lined baking dish, introduce in the oven at 680 degrees F and bake for 25 minutes

3   Slice into rectangle pieces when it gets cold and serve

Raspberry And Coconut

Ingredients:

- 2 cup swerve sweetener
- 2 cup coconut oil
- 2 cup raspberries; dried
- 2 cup coconut; shredded
- 2 cup coconut butter

Directions:

1. In your food processor, blend dried berries very well.
2. Heat a pan with the butter over medium heat.
3. Add oil, coconut and swerve; stir and cook for 10 minutes
4. Pour 2 of this into a lined baking pan and spread well.

5. Add raspberry powder and also spread.
6. Top with the rest of the butter mix, spread and keep in the fridge for a while
7. Cut into pieces and serve

Chocolate Pudding Delight

Ingredients:

- 2 teaspoon stevia powder
- 2 tablespoons cocoa powder
- 2 tablespoons water
- 2 tablespoon gelatin
- 2 cup of coconut milk
- 2 tablespoons maple syrup

Directions:

1. Heat a pan with the coconut milk over medium heat; add stevia and cocoa powder and mix well.
2. In a bowl, mix gelatin with water; stir well and add to the pan.

3. Stir well, add maple syrup, whisk again, divide into ramekins and keep in the fridge for 8 0 minutes Serve cold.

Peanut Butter Fudge

Ingredients:

- 2 cup almond milk
- 2 teaspoons vanilla stevia
- A pinch of salt
- 2 cup peanut butter; unsweetened
- 2 cup of coconut oil

For the topping:

- 2 cup cocoa powder
- 2 tablespoons melted coconut oil
- 2 tablespoons swerve sweetener

Directions:

1. In a heatproof bowl, mix peanut butter with 2 cup coconut oil; stir and heat up in your microwave until it melts
2. Add a pinch of salt, almond milk, and stevia; stir well everything and pour into a lined loaf pan.
3. Keep in the fridge for 2 hours and then slice it.
4. In a bowl, mix 2 tablespoons melted coconut with cocoa powder and swerve and stir very well.
5. Drizzle the sauce over your peanut butter fudge and serve

Cinnamon Streusel Fresh Egg Loaf

Ingredients:

- 2 tbsp grated butter, chilled
- 2 fresh egg
- 2 -ounce cream cheese
- 2 tbsp almond flour
- 2 tbsp butter, softened
- 2 tsp cinnamon, divided
- 2 tbsp erythritol sweetener, divided
- 2 tsp vanilla extract, unsweetened

Directions:

1. Turn on the oven, then set it to 680 degrees F and let it preheat.
2. Meanwhile, crack the fresh egg in a small bowl, add cream cheese, softened butter, 2 tsp cinnamon, 2 tbsp

sweetener, and vanilla and whisk until well combined.

3 Divide the fresh egg batter between two silicone muffins and then bake for 8 minutes.

4 Meanwhile, prepare the streusel and for this, place flour in a small bowl, add remaining ingredients and stir until well mixed.

5 When fresh egg loaves have baked, sprinkle streusel on top and then continue baking for 8 minutes.

6 When done, remove loaves from the cups, let them cool for 10 minutes and then serve and enjoy!

Snickerdoodle Muffins

Ingredients:

- 2 tbsp almond milk, unsweetened
- 2 tbsp erythritol sweetener and more for topping
- 2 tsp baking powder
- 2 tsp ground cinnamon and more for topping
- 2 tsp vanilla extract, unsweetened
- 2 tbsp coconut flour
- 2 of fresh egg
- 2 tbsp butter, unsalted, melted
- 2 tbsp whipping cream

Directions:

1 Turn on the oven, then set it to 680 degrees F and let it preheat.

2. Meanwhile, take a medium bowl, place flour in it, add cinnamon and baking powder. Stir until combined.
3. Take a separate bowl, place the 2 fresh egg in it, add butter, sour cream, milk, and vanilla and whisk until blended.
4. Whisk in flour mixture until a smooth batter is obtained, divide the batter evenly between two silicon muffin cups and then sprinkle cinnamon and sweetener on top.
5. Bake the muffins for 35to 35minutes until firm, and then the top has turned golden brown and then serve and enjoy!

Yogurt And Strawberry Bowl

Ingredients:

- 2 tbsp chopped walnuts
- 6 oz yogurt
- 6 oz mixed berries
- 2 tbsp chopped almonds

Directions:

1 Divide yogurt between two bowls, top with berries and then sprinkle with almonds and walnuts.
2 Serve and enjoy!

Sweet Cinnamon Muffin

Ingredients:

- 2 tsp erythritol sweetener
- 2 tsp baking soda
- 2 fresh fresh eggs
- 2 tsp coconut flour
- 2 tsp cinnamon

Directions:

1. Take a medium bowl, place all the ingredients in it, and whisk until well combined.
2. Take two ramekins, grease them with oil, distribute the prepared batter in it and then microwave for 2 minute and 8 0 seconds until done.

3 When done, take out muffin from the ramekin, cut in 2 , and then serve and enjoy!

Nutty Muffins

Ingredients:

- 2 tsp erythritol sweetener
- 2 fresh fresh egg   s
- 2 tsp almond butter, unsalted
- 6 tsp coconut flour
- 2 tsp baking soda

Directions:

1 Take a medium bowl, place all the ingredients in it, and whisk until well combined.
2 Take two ramekins, grease them with oil, distribute the prepared batter in it and

then microwave for 2 minute and 8 0 seconds until done.
3. When done, take out muffin from the ramekin, cut in 2 , and then serve and enjoy!

Pumpkin And Cream Cheese Cup

Ingredients:

- 2 of fresh egg
- 2 tbsp butter, unsalted
- 2 tsp pumpkin spice
- 2 tsp baking powder
- 2 tbsp erythritol sweetener
- 6 tbsp almond flour
- 2 tbsp coconut flour
- 2 tbsp pumpkin puree
- 2 tbsp cream cheese, softened

Directions:

1. Turn on the oven, then set it to 680 degrees F and let it preheat.
2. Take a medium bowl, place butter and 1 tbsp sweetener in it, and then beat until fluffy.
3. Beat in fresh egg and then beat in pumpkin puree until well combined.
4. Take a medium bowl, place flours in it, stir in pumpkin spice, baking powder until mixed, stir this mixture into the butter mixture and then distribute it into two silicone muffin cups.
5. Take a medium bowl, place cream cheese in it, and stir in remaining sweetener until well combined.
6. Divide the cream cheese mixture into the silicone muffin cups, swirl the batter and cream cheese mixture by using a toothpick and then bake for 35to 35minutes until muffins have turned firm.

7 Serve and enjoy!

Berries In Yogurt Cream

Ingredients:

- 2 ounce blackberries
- 2 ounce raspberry
- 2 tbsp erythritol sweetener
- 6 oz yogurt
- 6 oz whipping cream

Directions:

1. Take a medium bowl, place yogurt in it, and then whisk in cream.
2. Sprinkle sweetener over yogurt mixture, don't stir, cover the bowl with a lid, and then refrigerate for 2 hour.
3. When ready to serve, stir the yogurt mixture, divide it evenly between two

bowls, top with berries, and then serve and enjoy!

Pumpkin Pie Mug Cake

Ingredients:

- 2 tbsp whipping cream
- 2 fresh fresh egg   s
- 2 cup pumpkin puree
- 2 tbsp coconut flour
- 2 tsp sour cream

Others:

- 2 tsp cinnamon
- 2 tsp baking soda
- 2 tbsp erythritol sweetener

Directions:

1. Take a small bowl, place cream in it, and then beat in sweetener until well combined.
2. Cover the bowl, let it chill in the refrigerator for 80 minutes, then beat in fresh fresh eggs and pumpkin puree and stir in remaining ingredients until incorporated and smooth.
3. Divide the batter between two coffee mugs greased with oil and then microwave for 2 minutes until thoroughly cooked.
4. Serve and enjoy!

Chocolate And Strawberry Crepe

Ingredients:

- 2 fresh egg
- 2 tbsp coconut milk, unsweetened
- 2 tsp avocado oil
- 2 tsp baking powder
- 2 oz strawberry, sliced
- 2 tbsp coconut flour
- 2 tsp of cocoa powder
- 2 tsp flaxseed

Directions:

1 Take a medium bowl, place flour in it, and then stir in cocoa powder, baking powder, and flaxseed in it until mixed.
2 Add fresh egg and milk and then whisk until smooth.

3. Take a medium skillet pan, place it over medium heat, add 2 tsp oil and when hot, pour in 2 of the batter, spread it evenly, and then cook for 2 minute per side until firm.
4. Transfer crepe to a plate, add remaining oil, and cook another crepe by using the remaining batter.
5. When done, fill crepes with strawberries, fold them and then serve and enjoy!

Blackberry And Coconut Flour Cupcake

Ingredients:

- 2 fresh egg
- 2 ounce blackberry
- 2 tbsp butter, unsalted, chopped
- 2 tbsp erythritol sweetener
- 2 tsp baking powder
- 2 tsp vanilla extract, unsweetened
- 2 tbsp coconut flour
- 2 cup whipping cream
- 2 tbsp cream cheese

Directions:

1 Take a small bowl, place butter in it, add cream and them microwave for 60 to70

seconds until it melts, stirring every 25 seconds.
2. Then add cream cheese, cream, vanilla, and erythritol, whisk until smooth, whisk in coconut flour and baking powder until incorporated and then fold in berries.
3. Distribute the mixture evenly between four muffin cups, then bake for 35to 2 10 minutes until firm.
4. Serve and enjoy!

Coconut Soup

Ingredients:

- 2 -inch fresh ginger, peeled and grated
- 2 cup fresh cilantro, chopped
- Salt and ground black pepper to taste
- 2 tbsp fish sauce
- 2 tbsp coconut oil
- 2 tbsp mushrooms, chopped
- 6 oz shrimp, peeled and deveined
- 2 tbsp onion, chopped
- 2 tbsp fresh cilantro, chopped
- 6 cups of coconut milk
- 3 cups chicken stock
- 2 tsp fried lemongrass
- 6 lime leaves
- 6 Thai chilies, dried and chopped
- Juice from 2 lime

Directions:

1. In a medium pot, combine coconut milk, chicken stock, lemongrass, and lime leaves.
2. Preheat pot on medium heat.
3. Add Thai chilies, ginger, cilantro, salt, and pepper, stir and bring to simmer—Cook for 25 minutes.
4. Strain soup and return liquid to the pot.
5. Heat soup over medium heat.
6. Add fish sauce, coconut oil, mushrooms, shrimp, and onion. Stir well—Cook for 35minutes.
7. Add cilantro and lime juice, stir. Set aside for 35 minutes.
8. Serve.

Broccoli Soup

Ingredients:

- 2 cups vegetable stock
- 2 cup heavy cream
- Salt and ground black pepper to taste
- 2 tsp paprika
- 3 cups broccoli, divided into florets
- 2 cup cheddar cheese
- 2 cloves garlic
- 2 medium white fresh onion
- 2 tbsp butter
- 2 cups of water

Directions:

1. Peel and mince garlic. Peel and chop the onion.
2. Preheat pot on medium heat, add butter and melt it.

3 Add garlic and fresh onion and sauté for 6 minutes, stirring occasionally.
4 Pour in water, vegetable stock, heavy cream, and add pepper, salt, and paprika.
5 Stir and bring to boil.
6 Add broccoli and simmer for 4 0 minutes.
7 After that, transfer soup mixture to a food processor and blend well.
8 Grate cheddar cheese and add to a food processor, blend again.
9 Serve soup hot.

Simple Fresh Tomato Soup

Ingredients:

- 6 tbsp butter
- 2 tsp turmeric
- 2 oz red hot sauce
- Salt and ground black pepper to taste
- 6 tbsp olive oil
- 8 bacon strips, cooked and crumbled
- 8 oz fresh basil leaves, chopped
- 8 oz green fresh onions, chopped
- 6 cups canned fresh tomato soup
- 2 tbsp apple cider vinegar
- 2 tsp dried oregano

Directions:

1 Pour fresh tomato soup in the pot and preheat on medium heat. Bring to boil.

2. Add vinegar, oregano, butter, turmeric, hot sauce, salt, black pepper, and olive oil. Stir well.
3. Simmer the soup for 6 minutes.
4. Serve soup topped with crumbled bacon, green onion, and basil.

Green Soup

Ingredients:

- 2 cup spinach leaves
- 2 cup watercress
- 6 cups vegetable stock
- Salt and ground black pepper to taste
- 2 cup of coconut milk
- 2 cup parsley, for serving
- 2 cloves garlic
- 2 white fresh onion
- 2 cauliflower head
- 2 oz butter
- 2 bay leaf, crushed

Directions:

1. Peel and mince garlic. Peel and dice onion.
2. Divide cauliflower into florets.

3. Preheat pot on medium-high heat, add butter and melt it.
4. Add fresh onion and garlic, stir, and sauté for 6 minutes.
5. Add cauliflower and bay leaf, stir and cook for 6 minutes.
6. Add spinach and watercress, stir and cook for another 6 minutes.
7. Pour in vegetable stock—season with salt and black pepper. Stir and bring to boil.
8. Pour in coconut milk and stir well. Take off heat.
9. Use an immersion blender to blend well.
10. Top with parsley and serve hot.

Sausage And Peppers Soup

Ingredients:

- 6 oz canned jalapeños, chopped
- 6 oz canned fresh tomatoes, chopped
- 2 cup spinach
- 6 cups beef stock
- 2 tsp Italian seasoning
- 2 tbsp cumin
- 2 tsp fresh onion powder
- 2 tsp garlic powder
- 2 tbsp chili powder
- 2 tbsp avocado oil
- 2 lbs pork sausage meat
- Salt and ground black pepper to taste
- 2 green bell pepper, seeded and chopped

Directions:

1. Preheat pot with avocado oil on medium heat.
2. Put sausage meat in pot and brown for 10 minutes on all sides.
3. Add salt, black pepper, and green bell pepper and continue to cook for 6 minutes.
4. Add jalapeños and fresh tomatoes, stir well and cook for 2 minutes more.
5. Toss spinach and stir again close lid and cook for 8 minutes.
6. Pour in beef stock, Italian seasoning, cumin, fresh onion powder, chili powder, garlic powder, salt, and black pepper, stir well. Close lid again. Cook for 80 minutes.
7. When time is up, uncover the pot and simmer for 2 10 minutes more.
8. Serve hot.

Avocado Soup

Ingredients:

- 2 avocados, pitted, peeled, and chopped
- Salt and ground black pepper to taste
- ⅔ cup heavy cream
- 2 tbsp butter
- 2 scallions, chopped
- 6 cups chicken stock

Directions:

1. Preheat pot on medium heat, add butter and melt it.
2. Toss scallions, stir and sauté for 2 minutes.
3. Pour in 35 cups stock and bring to simmer—Cook for 6 minutes.
4. Meanwhile, peel and chop avocados.

5. Place avocado, 2 cup of stock, cream, salt, and pepper in a blender and blend well.
6. Add avocado mixture to the pot and mix well—Cook for 2 minutes.
7. Sprinkle with more salt and pepper, stir.
8. Serve hot.

Avocado And Bacon Soup

Ingredients:

- 2 tsp garlic powder
- Salt and ground black pepper to taste
- Juice of 2 lime
- 2 lb bacon, cooked and chopped
- 2 quart chicken stock
- 2 avocados, pitted
- 2 cup fresh cilantro, chopped

Directions:

1. Pour chicken stock in a pot and bring to boil over medium-high heat.
2. Meanwhile, peel and chop the avocados.
3. Place avocados, cilantro, garlic powder, salt, black pepper, and lime juice in

blender or food processor and blend well.
4 Add the avocado mixture in boiling stock and stir well.
5 Add bacon and season with salt and pepper to taste.
6 Stir and simmer for 5-10 minutes on medium heat.
7 Serve hot.

Roasted Bell Peppers Soup

Ingredients:

- 2 tbsp olive oil
- Salt and ground black pepper to taste
- 2 -quart chicken stock
- 2 cup water
- 2 cup Parmesan cheese, grated
- ⅔ cup heavy cream
- 2 medium white fresh onion
- 2 cloves garlic
- 2 celery stalks
- 3 oz roasted bell peppers, seeded

Directions:

1. Peel and chop fresh onion and garlic. Chop celery and bell pepper.
2. Preheat pot with oil on medium heat.

3. Put garlic, onion, celery, salt, and pepper in the pot, stir and sauté for 8 minutes.
4. Pour in chicken stock and water. Add bell peppers and stir.
5. Bring to boil, close lid, and simmer for 6 minutes. Reduce heat if needed.
6. When time is up, blend soup using an immersion blender.
7. Add cream and season with salt and pepper to taste. Take off heat.
8. Serve hot with grated cheese.

Spicy Bacon Soup

Ingredients:

- 2 cup cauliflower, divided into florets
- 6 oz green bell pepper, seeded and chopped
- 2 jalapeno pepper, seeded and chopped
- 6 cups chicken stock
- 2 tbsp full-fat cream
- 2 tsp ground black pepper
- 2 tsp chili pepper
- 2 oz bacon, chopped
- Salt to taste
- 2 tbsp olive oil

Directions:

1. In a bowl, combine bacon with salt.
2. Heat a pan over medium heat and cook bacon for 6 minutes, stirring constantly.

3 Remove bacon from pan and set aside.
4 Pour olive oil in a pan and add cauliflower, bell pepper, and jalapeno.
5 Cook vfresh egg ies on high heat for 2 minute, stirring occasionally.
6 In a saucepan, mix bacon with vegetables. Pour in chicken stock. Stir.
7 Close lid and cook for 40-45 minutes.
8 Open the lid and add cream, stir.
9 Season with salt, black pepper, and chili pepper. Stir and cook for 10 minutes more.
10 Serve.

Italian Sausage Soup

Ingredients:

- 8 cups chicken stock
- 2 lb radishes, chopped
- 2 oz spinach
- 2 cup heavy cream
- 6 bacon slices, chopped
- Salt and ground black pepper to taste
- A pinch of red pepper flakes
- 2 tsp avocado oil
- 2 cloves garlic
- 2 medium white fresh onion
- 3 lbs hot pork sausage, chopped

Directions:

1. Preheat pot on medium-high heat and add oil.
2. Peel and chop garlic and onion.

3. Put garlic, onion, and sausage in the pot and stir.
4. Cook for few minutes until browned.
5. Pour in chicken stock; add radishes and spinach, stir.
6. Bring mixture to simmer and add cream, bacon, black pepper, salt, and red pepper flakes, stir well.
7. Simmer for 25 minutes.
8. Serve hot.

Cabbage Hash Browns

Ingredients

- 2 slices of bacon
- 2 tsp garlic powder
- 2 fresh egg
- 2 cup shredded cabbage

Seasoning:

- 2 tbsp coconut oil
- 2 tsp salt
- 2 tsp ground black pepper

Directions:

1. Crack the fresh egg in a bowl, add garlic powder, black pepper, and salt, whisk well, then add cabbage, toss until well mixed and shape the mixture into four patties.

2. Take a fresh skillet pan, place it over medium heat, add oil and when hot, add patties in it and cook for 10 minutes per side until golden brown.
3. Transfer hash browns to a plate, then add bacon into the pan and cook for 10 minutes until crispy.
4. Serve hash browns with bacon.

Cauliflower Hash Browns

Ingredients

- 2 tsp garlic powder
- 2 fresh   fresh egg   white
- 1/2   cup grated cauliflower
- 2 slices of bacon

Seasoning:

- 2 tsp salt
- 2   tsp ground black pepper
- 2 tbsp coconut oil

Directions:

1. Place grated cauliflower in a heatproof bowl, cover with plastic wrap, poke some holes in it with a fork and then microwave for 10 minutes until tender.
2. Let steamed cauliflower cool for 35minutes, then wrap in a cheesecloth

and squeeze well to drain moisture as much as possible.

3. Crack the fresh egg in a bowl, add garlic powder, black pepper, and salt, whisk well, then add cauliflower and toss until well mixed and sticky mixture comes together.

4. Take a fresh skillet pan, place it over medium heat, add oil and when hot, drop cauliflower mixture on it, press lightly to form hash brown patties, and cook for 5 to 10 minutes per side until browned.

5. Transfer hash browns to a plate, then add bacon into the pan and cook for 10 minutes until crispy.

6. Serve hash browns with bacon.

www.ingramcontent.com/pod-product-compliance
Lightning Source LLC
LaVergne TN
LVHW011943070526
838202LV00054B/4773